THE SCIENCE OF ACHIEVING
GREATNESS

Level Up Your Life For A Big Game, Unleash Your

Hidden Potential To Create Abundance, Scientifically

Shirish Kawthale

www.Shirishkawthale.com

Copyright and Disclaimer

All rights reserved. © Shirish Kawthale 2021

No portion of this book shall be used or may be replicated, transmitted, downloaded, decompiled, or stored any form or by any means, whether electronic or mechanical, photocopying, recording, without the express written permission of the publisher.

The publisher and the author would like to apologize for any missing acknowledgments and will be pleased to incorporate them in any future edition of this book.

The author, as well as the publisher, shall not be held liable or responsible to any person for any loss or harm caused or alleged to have been caused, directly or indirectly, resulting out of the use of the information from this book. The intention of the author is only to offer information of general nature. If you use any of the information in this book for yourself, the author does not assume responsibility for your action.

The author shall not be liable whatsoever for any errors, omissions, whether such errors or omissions result from negligence or by accident, and for the reliability, accuracy, or sufficiency of the information.

Dedication

DEDICATED TO, NITIN...
MY BROTHER,
MY BEST FRIEND,
WHO WAS ALWAYS WITH ME
UNCONDITIONALLY...

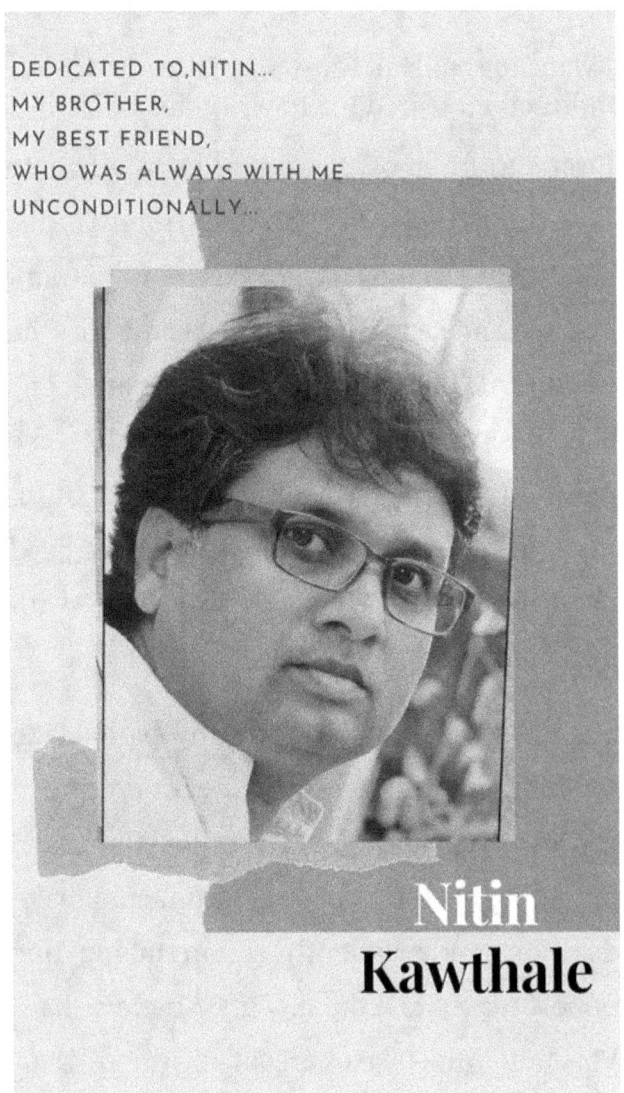

Nitin Kawthale

Acknowledgment

I want to thank all those who directly or indirectly inspired me to write this book.

First and foremost, I would like to attribute my whole life to my three spiritual Gurus. The first among the three is Swami Vivekananda, who introduced me to the world of spirituality. The second my Gnyaneshwar Mauli made me realize the truth and introduced me to my third Guru, my Lord Krishna, whom I believe once lived on this planet as a human being with unbound potential.

I attribute my whole life to my parents, to my Mother, Mrs.Saraswati, for everything in my life. My Father, Mr. Digambar Kawthale, for giving me the freedom to think and make decisions independently. I am taking this opportunity to thank my better half, Vaishali, who takes care of me more than myself and my son Atharva for bringing tons of love and happiness into my life and the desire to live, and without his support, this book wouldn't have been written.

I also want to thank my Uncle, Mr.Dattatray Kawthale, who has been holding my hand since childhood. My brother Nitin kawthale, to whom I have dedicated my book. I want to thank all the Kawthale family members who are truly outstanding.

I want to mention the names of my friends who are more than friends to me. First, Ashok Bhale, my childhood friend, with whom I love to spend time, and Gangadhar Rudrurkar, my schoolmate, gave me the real joy of true friendship and intimacy. Mr.Balaji Gajewar and Mr.Balaji Zampalkar are the two of my friends with whom I enjoyed my life most.

Finally, I want to thank all the beautiful people who helped me to become me as I am today.

Contents

Copyright and Disclaimer......3

Acknowledgment......6

Contents......8

Introduction......10

Know your brain to unlock the abundance......19

The Science of Thinking Right......26

Affirmations that work like magic......41

Visualization; designing the future......51

The ultimate science of Belief......60

Perception; the ultimate solution to all problems......71

Character, the foundation for Achieving Greatness..................77

The Science of Habit..........................98

Self-image, the man in the mirror............................108

Goal setting; setting the sail..117

Action -The only key to success....................................124

Time; the principal asset for achieving greatness...............130

Knowing the facts of life, essential for achieving greatness.................135

Recipe for achieving Greatness..157

Introduction

When I was in school, I was an average student. I never studied. My mind never got interested in the subjects taught in the school. What I could understand was only my emotions and love towards my family and friends. As a child, I was highly devoted to my friends and sports.

When I was in the tenth standard, one day, my science teacher asked me, "what are MKS and CGS ?" I was there in the middle of the classroom, and all eyes were staring at me. I was extremely baffled and completely blank. The words were entirely unknown to me. I felt those two words, like the two atom bombs, thrown by America on Hiroshima and Nagasaki during the second world war. Those words confounded me. I was speechless, and extremely nervous.

And my teacher kept asking me about the SI units of measurement. Being in the tenth standard, he was expecting me to talk something about it. I was trying to avoid his eye contact because I could never forget the way he looked at me. Looking at his expressions, I could feel as if I was not from this planet.

After the tenth's result, one of my close friends suggested me to focus on the studies and become a doctor, as the friend was very close to me, could believe in me. I had taken the words very seriously. And for the first time in my life, I had started to study hard and began to think about my life and career.

Somehow, I could score 95 marks in Biology but couldn't perform well in other subjects and failed to fulfill the expectations.

It was the first major failure in my life. Till the results, I was on cloud nine, and the moment the result came, I was all upset. I didn't want to meet anyone, face anyone and give any excuse for my failure. If truth be told, I tried to run away from home. I had filled my bag with all my documents and reached the bus stop. I waited for the bus. On that day, all I wanted to escape from that situation so that nobody could ask me about my result.

The bus didn't come on time. I had to wait a long there. As the time was passing very slow that day, I was feeling afraid of being confronted with someone familiar. Finally, when the bus arrived, I saw one of my friends had arrived at the bus stand. I had no other option except to talk with him. Though I didn't reveal my real motive for being there, my conversation with him had drained all my courage. I just spent some time with him there and came back home.

Since I was very disappointed and didn't want to talk with anyone, I didn't put a single step out of my house for a whole one month. It was like self-imposed imprisonment.

That was the most critical period of my life. I was completely depressed, turned introvert, and started thinking a lot.

Fortunately, I had found the complete volumes of Swami Vivekananda's philosophy. When I was reading his philosophy, I found it most appealing to me. I was totally immersed in reading his thoughts about life and the truth. During the same period, I found Gnyaneshwari, which literally changed my life. This book is the commentary on Bhagavad-Gita, the best book ever in Marathi by Saint Gnyaneshwar, one of the eminent saints of Maharashtra. I was resonating with the thoughts and the philosophy of Vivekananda and Bhagavad-Gita. I could feel it as it was all written for me. Their views had changed my perspective of life.

But my failure in becoming a doctor had deeply hurt me. It never allowed me to remain quiet. No matter what, I wanted to achieve success. So, I kept on trying, never gave up. Then I tried for the civil services exam and failed. I tried my luck in network marketing, and I again failed. Every time I failed, my desire to achieve success became more aggravated. So, I was desperate to find success.

So, I started reading a lot, thinking a lot about success. I read several self-help books, numerous case studies, along with reading science and philosophy books. My condition at that period is rightly described in Emily Dickinson's poem, "success is counted sweetest."

Success is counted sweetest,

By those who never succeed.

> To comprehend the nectar,
>
> Requires the sorest need.

But, even if had I achieved any of my goals, I wouldn't have settled down with it. The impact of the thoughts of Vivekananda and the Bhagavad-Gita on me was so profound. I had a complete transformation from within. My perspective of life had changed entirely. I wanted to give a wholesome response to life's calling. I wanted to lead a more meaningful life. That's why I couldn't match myself with the goals I was setting for myself. And I couldn't focus 100% on any goal since a part of me was always in search of something more meaningful, something more than mere success.

So far, I had learned that all great people are successful, but not all successful people are great. Hence, the concept of achieving greatness intrigued my mind. I think greatness is something more and rare, and to be great is a unique thing. It gives you a distinct identity, apart from the crowd. To be great is the quality of a rare breed.

Successful people are remembered for some time, but the great people are simply unforgettable.

After years of study, I realized that there is a science behind achieving greatness, and I realized that this science could transform any ordinary person into an extraordinary person.

At this present moment, I have nothing great achievements to share with you except my **conviction** in the principles, which I will unfold to you in the chapters of this book. This conviction has come to me as the result of my past 25 years of research, my relentless search for a meaningful life, many sleepless nights, total restless journey, and numerous long lonely walks contemplating, analyzing, evaluating each aspect of my life.

I promise you, with my conviction, that you will be all on your path to achieving greatness when you will finish the book. You will find the acres of Diamond under your feet. You will find yourself the master of your destiny. You will feel empowered to design your future. With my book, you will be able to bring that abundance to your life and sustain it.

Each chapter in this book will bring that insight to you. The chapters have been placed in the order of their significance in the way of achieving greatness. But each chapter is equally potent to bring that change in you, which can transform your life.

The principles I talked about in this book are all based on scientific truths. They will work for each one of you irrespective of your present status quo, provided you should absorb the message and act upon it.

I believe the readers of my book will appreciate my efforts to add value to their lives. And I am pretty sure my science teacher will be thrilled at the sight of my book on the science of achieving greatness.

I will be immensely pleased and will eagerly be waiting for your comments and suggestions.

Let's begin our journey of self-transformation for achieving greatness by learning about the miraculous human brain and its immense potential.

Chapter 1

Know your brain to unlock the abundance

Since the beginning of human evolution, from the moment the first human being existed on this planet and from the day when the transformation of his life from beast to modern-day civilized man began, and the day when he discovered the wheel- which marked the beginning of his progress, that he has made till today in various fields like science and technology, health, education, transport, and business not only in society at a national and global level but also in space, almost everything he has achieved so far must be attributed to the human brain.

With the brain, everything exists, and without a brain, nothing would have existed.

This human brain is what scientists call the most unique and complex organ on this planet, a three-pound universe, creator, and destroyer at the same time.

Creations like languages, culture, traditions, values, the whole civilization; everything was possible for the human being only because of the brain.
Although we as humans are not far different from the rest of the living beings. We, too, are dependent on this nature for survival. From the humanistic point of view, we are also the creations of this nature.

This nature, you may call it the creator, has given all the living beings something special, unique to protect themselves and survive. But this nature has given nothing to humans except this fantastic brain. Only because of that, man could develop himself from his original primitive beastlike state to a modern-day civilized man. In contrast, we can see the rest of the animals are still in their primitive state.

So, why is our brain so amazing? Even modern scientists have still not found out all the mysteries of our brain. It has been surprising them for ages.

Our brain, though, weighs only 2% of our body's weight but consumes 20% of the total supply of oxygen and energy. It can produce 23 watts of power when awake, with which we can light a lamp in the house. There are nearly 100000 miles of tiny blood vessels that carry almost one litre of blood per minute.

This brain is made of approx. 100 billion neuron cells equal to the stars in our galaxy or the leaves in the Amazon jungle. The size of each neuron cell is 4 microns, which means we can fit tens of thousands of neuron cells on the tip of a pin. Each neuron cell is capable of making approx. 40000 synapses and sends nearly 1000 neuro impulses per second. These synapses are the seat of information, 100 billion in number. Each can make up to 40000 synapses, which means an incredibly huge amount of information (in Petabytes) can be stored in these quadrillion connections.

Every human's brain has equal potential. It performs approx. 60 trillion actions per second. Controlling blood pressure, maintain body temperature, and keeping the heartbeats are some of the most flabbergasting activities which the brain performs. It can identify 10000 different smells. It works faster than the supercomputer.

Besides this, the brain is the head chemist in our body. It secretes hormones, essential chemicals in the blood as a response to our Perception. The chemicals it releases are serotonin, oxytocin, endorphin, and dopamine, which are positive chemicals. As dopamine is a happy drug, it makes you feel good. Endorphin fills you with energy, enthusiasm. Oxytocin builds your self-esteem and bonds you with your partner. It also releases cortisol, the stress hormone, which creates an immediate response to threats, switches the body in flight or fight mode as a part of a survival mechanism.

Though all human beings have the same physical brain, we can see that all have different IQs, but the surprising fact about IQ is that it mostly depends on the state of mind and the level of brainwaves. The brain remains at varying levels of brainwaves at different times. When we are in a deep sleep, it is in delta waves. Before falling asleep and waking up from sleep, it remains in theta wave for a few minutes. When awake, it is in alpha level, and when we are wide awake and active, it is in Beta wave.

It is now well known that the physical brain is the hardware and the mind being the software, rules the body. This mind is 5% conscious and 95% subconscious. This conscious mind is creative and has free will, but the subconscious mind is programmed. It decides our fate by controlling our habits if we don't do anything about it.

Modern-day sciences like Neuroplasticity, Epigenetic, Neuroscience, and quantum physics have brought into light new aspects of the human brain. That has opened a new world of opportunities empowering us to write our destiny on our own.

Knowing the brain itself will be the Game Changer.

Mind being the software of the brain, and the governor of this body controls the operations of the brain like thinking, Perception, beliefs, habits, and holds and carries the software of our personality, which becomes our self-image.

Therefore, it becomes highly essential to know the nature of all these mind's operations for achieving greatness. So, we will start with the primary function of our brain, i.e., thinking. Let's dive deep into the science of thinking in the next chapter.

Chapter 2

The Science of Thinking Right

Cogito, ergo sum. *"I think; therefore, I am."*   Rene Descartes

The spontaneous flow of thoughts in the human mind is the proof of our existence, as Rene states in his Principles of Philosophy. Thinking is associated with the neurotransmissions in the brain, which pass through the different synapses. It is estimated that we have nearly 70 thousand thoughts per day. Out of this, almost 75 % of thoughts are repetitive. And unfortunately, most of them are negative.

Now, it's been well known that the human body is made of 60 trillion cells. Each cell has its brain. And mind, being the governor of the body, there is constant communication between mind and body. The community of 60 trillion cells knows, every single moment, what's going on in mind. Every single thought, every single word it utters, signals the body and which starts manifesting it.

In the 1960's Dr. Roger Sperry got the Nobel prize for his work on the Split-brain theory. According to him, our human brain has two hemispheres, the left, and the right. These two hemispheres are connected with the corpus callosum, which is made of 300 million nerve fibers and works as the bridge between the two hemispheres. Though these two hemispheres work distinctively and have been assigned different functions, they synchronize the information. The left brain is the Auditory system, works on language, and the Right-brain controls the visuals. As we know, we receive 83 % of our knowledge through our eyes. The occipital lobe covers almost 20 % of our brain size. That's why we remember the faces and forget the names of people.

So, when the mind thinks, the right brain starts picturizing it. It creates images relevant to the thoughts. As per the pictures in mind, the brain starts secreting the chemicals. When we think negatively, thoughts of fears, doubts overpower us, and we feel like in stress, and the brain starts secreting cortisol, a stress hormone, which creates flight or fight mode in the body, either to fight with the situation or to fly away from it. So, the blood is supplied more to the arms and limbs to fight or to run. In the lack of enough supply of blood, the brain narrows down its focus. That's why we make silly mistakes when we are in tension. If the stress continues for an extended period, it reduces the body's immune system, and these people find themselves caught in some disease. The word Disease itself means **dis-ease,** not at comfort. As the old African proverb says," *If there is no enemy within, the enemy outside can do us no harm."*

The science behind Buddha's Quote- What you think you become.

In Modern sciences, Epigenetics studies the factors that affect gene activity. Dr. Bruce Lipton, the cell biologist, has done remarkable research in this field. According to him, your genetic activity is controlled by the chemistry of the blood.

The human brain, being the head chemist in our body, secretes the chemicals in the blood. The blood is the environment of the cell. The type of chemical it secretes depends on the kind of thoughts in our mind. If you think of some problem and the ideas of fear, worry, and doubt prevail in your mind, the right brain starts creating similar images. As a result, the brain perceives the threat and starts secreting the stress hormone cortisol to prepare the body to face the situation. If the thoughts are of anger, excitement, and anxiety, then the brain secretes adrenaline, and if your mind is filled with love, care, and sympathy, the blood is supplied with oxytocin and serotonin. When your mind is filled with a sense of fulfillment and is happy, then endorphin and dopamine are released in the blood. And the most crucial part is that, if the situation persists for a long, our body gets habituated with that particular chemical. It gets addicted. So, the body manifests the circumstances to receive that specific chemical again and again. Therefore, we can see that people live throughout their life carrying the same baggage of their sorrows, worries, fears, and some carry their happiness and joy. So, at the root, your thoughts lead the brain to secrete the chemicals, and the genes, in turn, manifest it into reality.

According to Quantum physics, our consciousness creates our reality. All our experiences are the result of all our thinking and what's going on inside our brains. And these experiences, the environment are again programming our mind, body, and our destiny.

Quantum physics states that everything is in the form of energy. Everything is in the form of vibration. Our thoughts are also in the form of vibrations. As per the law of attraction, similar vibes attract. So, your thoughts attract things with similar vibrations. Unfortunately, your 75 % thoughts are repetitive and are mostly negative ones, so people live in the same circumstances throughout their life.

The science of positive thinking.

"*The quality of happiness in your life depends on the quality of your thoughts.*" Marcus Aurelius.

Now it is pretty clear that why positive thinking works like magic. When we think positive, when we think of success, think of happiness and joy, the brain creates the relevant positive images and releases growth hormones like endorphins, oxytocin, serotonin, and dopamine. So, everything goes well, the body's homeostasis is maintained, and the brain gets enough oxygen and energy. Mind being happy and at comfort, thinks clearly, makes better choices, makes better decisions, gets better results, and becomes more comfortable and healthier.

Positive thinking involves the use of positive words as the words are the instruments of thoughts. Positive words help the brain to create positive images, and the cycle goes on. That's why it was found in a survey that most highly successful people have a vast vocabulary. Having enriched vocabulary helps them use the right words, which creates the correct pictures in mind, and with the right images, they get the right results.

So, I call these positive words the success vocabulary. Indeed, the words have magical powers. Therefore, I have given the name of this topic as the science of thinking right. Thinking right in a sense, thinking with correct words. So, thinking right can make you strong, powerful, happy, and successful. These thoughts can make you healthy, wealthy, and famous. At the same time, if you ignore right-thinking, your thoughts can bring you poverty, weakness, and defame. Your thoughts can make your life miserable. Using the right words is the key to all positive thinking. For instance, when we say,

I will try to achieve it or finish something. The mind perceives it as **trying** that is more important than attaining or completing, and it creates the pictures of trying, not the images of achieving or accomplishments. So, people who say, I will try, seldom achieve success. And so, just by using the right words, you can change your life.

Human thoughts are connected; they have their entity. Thoughts do have some power. If we think of telepathy, we can know that all our human minds are connected. I will tell you an incident in support of the above statement, which Swami Vivekananda mentioned in his writing.

Once, Swamiji had gone to visit a mystic saint at a remote place with his disciples. The saint was known for reading the minds of people. When people came to that saint, he would ask the people to write anything on a piece of paper and fold the paper, and then the saint used to tell the people what was written on that piece of paper without looking into it. So Swamiji wanted to test his skill and wrote sentences in a different language, which the mystic saint easily read without looking into it.

Swamiji also mentioned that, in his later years, when his disciples would come to ask him anything, he would answer their questions in advance, well before being asked by his disciples and letting them remain surprised.

I want to mention one more incident which took place in Australia, where a large group of people were asked to send the energy to the seeds and later it was found that these charged seeds grew faster than the regular seeds. You might have also heard about the Japanese Dr. Masaru Emoto's experiment showing the impact of thoughts on rice and water. By giving these examples, I just wanted to bring to you that our thoughts really do have some power that can affect external things. Some of you might agree with me that when our mother cooks food, it tastes more delicious. Only because of this influence of thoughts on the external world can we believe to some extent that ancient Indian saints really might have exercised the mystical power of Chanting Mantras. They could exercise that power only because they would live what they think, say, and do. Their thoughts, words, and their actions used to be in complete alignment.

All of us experience this at some point in our lives when we find ourselves in the midst of fear, doubt, confusion and remain clueless on how to get out of this. We go to a temple, church, or Mosque, and we pray to our God. What happens when we pray? We feel our mind becomes calm, it seeks some unknown assurance, and suddenly some idea pops up, revealing the solution to our problem. It happens because when we pray, we can access the universal infinite intelligence. So somewhere we are all connected, our thoughts are connected.

And in this perspective, I find the statement made by Charles Haanel, a quantum physicist, very appropriate. He states- *"There is but one consciousness of which your consciousness must be a part, must be the same in kind and quality as a whole, the difference being one of degree."*

The magical words... Abracadabra

We hear these words when we see a magician performing and trying to bring something surprising. Actually, the words are in the Hebrew language, which means, **What I think is what I create**. Isn't it surprising that Buddha also told the same thing when he says, *"What you think you become, what you feel you attract and what you imagine you create."* Indeed, our mind is like a magic wand. Whatever you hold in your mind, it grows. The thoughts in your mind create your reality. Consequently, you are what you think about.

James Allen rightly said it in different words. He stated, *"The circumstances don't make a man; they reveal him."*

I will conclude this chapter by telling you a story of a great leader from Indian history. Some of you might know his name. The story I am going to tell you is of Lokmanya Bal Gangadhar Tilak, who is known as the Father of Indian unrest, during India's freedom struggle.

Tilak was born in the period of India's first freedom struggle. During that period, Tilak's Grandfather was in Kashi, the Hindu religious place in North India, where the major uprisings happened. He had witnessed the struggle closely.

When Tilak was learning in primary school, he used to rush to his Grandfather immediately after school. His Grand Father would tell him the stories of great Indian freedom fighters who fought bravely against British rule and devoted their whole life to the motherland. These Stories deeply impacted and sowed the thoughts of making India free from British rule, intensely in his mind. And the rest is history.

In short, your thoughts create your reality. Use them wisely. Every second, they are in the process of molding your life. I know all of us can't have control over the spontaneous flow of thoughts. But we have a formidable solution for this in the next chapter. Let's jump in and check it.

Chapter 3

Affirmations that work like magic

The quality of your self-talk determines the level of your life.   Shirish.

By the dictionary meaning, to affirm means to declare something as true to yourself. It is now well known that our minds and body are in constant communication. Every single thought that comes into your mind signals the whole body, and the 60 trillion cells respond accordingly.

Neuroplasticity is the human brain's ability to form new neural paths as a result of learning, change in environment, or stress, and many other factors. Earlier it was believed that this neuroplasticity was possible only in the brain of children. And the brain of an adult is unchanged, but in the latter half of 20th century, discoveries in neuroscience and research on the human brain brought into light the new aspects of the human brain. It was discovered that the human brain is malleable and can be rewired at any point in time.

Strong, positive affirmations really work like wonders, and they make new connections and new neural paths. They can bring the desired change in the behavior, in the understanding and the attitude of a person.

Focused brain

We know that nearly 60 thousand thoughts come into our minds every day. We can't control or stop these thoughts, but we can direct these thoughts by positive affirmations. Our brain has a unique character. It is very focused. It usually finds out what is asked to find and search. When you feel hungry and are walking through the market, your brain automatically finds out the spots and brings forth the places where you can feed yourself. So, with strong positive affirmations, we can set the focus and direction of the brain on our desired change. It is like reprogramming our subconscious brain with conscious desires.

Our mind is 5% creative, conscious, and 95% programmed subconscious, and is a habit brain. All the beliefs, habits, and behavior come under the control of our subconscious mind, and unfortunately, we get this programming before the age of 7. We don't have any control over it. We can't choose our programming at that age. But with strong positive affirmations, a burst of new chemical reactions starts in our brain that changes the old neural paths and creates the new pathways that align with our conscious desires.

Throughout the day, the brain passes through the different states of brain waves.

Different state of brainwaves represents the different levels of awareness or consciousness. When we are in a deep sleep, our brain remains in the state of delta waves. Before falling asleep and immediately after getting awake, it passes through the state of theta waves, which is the hypnotic state, when the subconscious mind is open and ready to receive the new programming. When we are awake, our brain stays in the state of Alfa waves, which is very conducive for learning. When we are wide awake and in a very active mode, our brain remains in the state of beta waves during the daytime.

In the book of Job, in verse no.33:15:16, It is told, "*In a dream, in a vision of the night,*

> *When deep sleep falls upon men,*
>
> *Whilest slumbering on their beds,*
>
> *Then he opens the ears of men ,*
>
> *And seals their instructions ."*

So, what we think, what we hear, in the last few minutes before we go to bed, before we fall asleep are the things we place in our subconscious mind. Negative self-talk at this time really ruins our life.

This is the most crucial time of the day you should use to reprogram your mind.

The present tense brain

Though made of 100 billion neuron cells, with quadrillion connections, and performing trillions of actions per sec, the human brain can't differentiate between past, future, and present. Everything that happens is happening at this moment for our brain. Whatever we think about the past or future, the brain prepares our body to respond in the present moment of thinking. The moment you decide to do something exciting in the future, for example, when you decide to meet someone very dear to you,

you start feeling excited now. When we plan for our summer trip, though well in advance, we start feeling excited now. The students who prepare for the exam and can't focus on their studies start feeling nervous at the thought of taking exams. Our brain responds to our thoughts in the present moment.

Therefore, our affirmations must be in the present tense. If you tell yourself," I will be studying hard for my future exams.' Then the brain prepares your body to undergo that hardship now and not in the future. Instead of that, if you say," I love to study hard." that strengthens the new connections in the brain that makes you prepare easily at the time of exams.

The positive brain

The human brain can't understand the negative command. Unfortunately, since our childhood, we have been given negative orders. Even today, we too provide negative commands to our kids and friends. For example, when we give or listen to a command like, Don't worry, Don't do it, Don't shout, Don't cry. Our brain starts processing the order and listens to the main verb worry or shout, or cry and prepares our body to react, and at the same time, it starts working on the don't command and starts negating the entire preparation to act upon. But as we don't give or receive the exact instruction of what to be done, our brain remains confused and ends up doing the exact opposite of what we expect. Hence, instead of saying, I am not afraid of anything, we must say, I am brave.

Some of the other things we need to consider before using affirmations to bring the desired change are

1. Personal affirmations.

Every person is unique in this world with a distinctive character, exclusive personality.

He/she has a different set of beliefs and experiences. So, it is always better to make our personal affirmations. They work fast, easy to believe, and can be more relevant.

2. The power of the pen.

Writing the affirmations on paper gives extra benefits. When we write on paper, we think and write with hand, which profoundly impacts our mind. We use Auditory cognitive skills when we think and say the affirmation in our mind. We also use visual cognitive skills when we see what's written and use kinesthetic skills too. When we use different cognitive skills, for one thing, it makes a more profound imprint on the mind.

3. Use of technology.

Today, everybody has got smartphones. These phones have tones of applications, which are helpful and are equally effective. We should make the most use of it.

4. Use the affirmations before going to bed.

It indeed works 100%. But we need to take care. We should be using positive words and use only the present tense. Never go for extreme affirmations. They must be realistic. Listen affirmations at least once a week before going to bed.

In Vedanta philosophy, the practitioners are asked to repeat the Mahavakyas every day and affirm them repeatedly throughout the day. Mahavakyas are the sentences of ultimate truth like Aham brahmasmi, Tatvamasi.

Aham Brahmasmi means I am the Ultimate Soul, and Tatvamasi implies that you are the ultimate truth. It is the highest form of affirmations. Indians have been using it for ages.

I hope you got the message, right! Self-talk, Auto suggestions, Affirmations, call it by any name, is the magic stick with which you can indeed bring magical change in your life.

In the next chapter, I will be talking about one of the most influential faculty of our brain, with which you can bring any desired change just by lying in a bed. Curious to know, then don't wait. Just keep reading. I have an abundance of secrets ready to reveal...

Chapter 4

Visualization; designing the future

Imagination is more powerful than Knowledge.

Albert Einstein.

Visualization is the mind's ability to create images and visuals. When added with emotions and feelings, it works like magic. This quality of visualizing can be the most creative as well as destructive. To use it constructively for positive results, we have to operate this brain's ability wisely. But the mind uses this power of visualization for negative things without our conscious efforts. When we are afraid of something, it's because of the mind's negative imagination. When we are worried, the mind is busy visualizing the negative pictures of possible outcomes.

When emotions get added to these visualizations, it seriously impacts overall physical and mental health. Positive and optimistic visualization with feelings of joy and fulfillment create wonders, and negative and pessimistic visualization with emotions of fear and guilt can equally worsen the situation.

As we discussed earlier, though our brain has enormous potential, it can't differentiate between reality and imagination and between the Past, Future, and Present. It responds to real and imaginary situations alike. It can be better understood if we can recall our experience of watching a movie in a theatre. We have the swing of emotions as the story goes on, the events in the film make us laugh, make us feel sad, sometimes make us angry, and we do cry sometimes. It also happens with us when we are sleeping and dreaming. We feel angry, scared and sometimes we weep in dreams.

The thing I want to tell you is that we can fool our brains. Yes, it's 100% true. And this secret is now not a secret since People have been using this for a long time. Artists and Athletes use it to improve their performance.

A famous example is of fourth World chess champion Alexander Alekhine, who defeated his earlier world chess champion Capablanca. Everybody was favoring Capablanca as he was undefeated. Alekhine had never won against Capablanca.

It has been said that Alekhine used his technical skills and wild imagination to defeat the unbeaten Capablanca. Alekhine could do this because, when he was in school, at the age of 12, he could analyze his chess game during school hours, sitting in a classroom, without a chessboard, all in his head, imagining and visualizing. He had started playing chess blindfolded. He was a Russian, and during the first world war, he was found playing chess in Germany and was caught and imprisoned. In prison, he had no newspapers, no books, and no chessboard too. He used to play chess in his imagination, just visualizing. In 1924 he made a new world record of playing blindfolded against 28 players.

In 1927, before the world championship, Alekhine had researched the Capablanca's game and found his weakness and had practiced using his imaginations and defeated Capablanca many times in his visualization. When Alekhine defeated Capablanca and became the World chess champion, and the entire chess world was surprised.

Not only Alekhine but Muhammad Ali, Mike Tyson, and the greatest Olympic champion of all time, Michael Phelps, used high-level visualization techniques. Moreover, Tyson would go to his night visualization routine almost every day before going to bed.

There are several other examples of research done on studying the effect of visualization. In one incident, a group of music learners was divided into two groups. One group was asked to practice with the musical instrument, and the other was asked to practice in mind by visualizing; later, after few days, it was found that the progress made by both the groups was not significantly different. When athletes were asked to carry their work out in mind, just by imagining, It was found that they took the same amount of time, and they, in fact, got exhausted.

Why visualization works

The human brain has unique and distinctive qualities. One of such distinct characteristics of the brain is, it loves comfort. There is an autopilot programming in the brain that always tries to keep us safe and avoid pain. It also tries to save energy and time, all as a part of an automated survival mechanism.

When we plan something big and prepare ourselves to go for it, we do it with our conscious mind, which is only 5%. Our 95% brain is a habit brain whose primary role is to keep us safe and avoid pain. When we set ourselves for the big task, this brain looks at the big task ahead, makes the calculations, and finds it consuming more energy and time, and it doesn't want to lose its comfort. Brain, as we have seen, stays in the present; it responds in the present. It loves the familiarity. Now the brain has got habituated itself with the present and is comfortable with it. So even though we try to push ourselves hard with our 5% conscious brain, we usually fail to sustain our progress after few days.

But when we visualize that big task and imagine it vividly, making aware and familiar with each aspect of it and start thinking and behaving as if we have achieved it. With enough of this practice, our brain gets that familiarity. It makes itself comfortable with the new surroundings, even though that surrounding or situation exists only in our mind. We know that it can't differentiate between reality and imagination. When athletes have enough of this visualization, it helps them be at comfort at the actual time of competition, killing that anxiety.

Besides this, when this visualization is coupled with emotions, it creates a ripple effect. As visualizing with emotions make that imprint on the subconscious mind, and the law of attraction works. It attracts similar vibes. And we can see whatever we have envisioned turning into reality.

Dr.Victor Frankl, in his book, The man's search for meaning, wrote about his experiences when he was in a Nazi concentration camp. He alone was the survivor from his family. Later wrote a book. He mentioned that those who had a strong purpose could visualize intensely, develop longevity, and survive.

Visualizing, creating pictures is a part of the right-brain activity. As the images are more powerful than words, as we remember the faces and usually forget the names, pictures in mind make a substantial impact. They work as the lighthouse, direct our minds, send a clear message to the whole body. If we remain aware of our unconscious negative visualization and replace it with the desired future images, our subconscious mind will do the rest.

Well, I hope you have understood the power of visualization. I would suggest you make a habit of visualizing every day before going to bed. Else you can make your vision board and place it just right in front of your bed so that you can watch it every night before falling asleep.

In the next chapter, I will discuss the power of belief and the science behind it.

Chapter 5

The ultimate science of Belief

Our brain is the hardware and the mind being the software, 5% conscious and 95% subconscious. A conscious mind is creative, has free will, can decide and learn new things, gets motivated, and plans for the future. However, the subconscious is a programmed mind. It is a habit brain. Beliefs and habits come under the control of this Subconscious mind.

Beliefs are the thoughts we have accepted as true. We create these beliefs after experiencing certain things, and most of the beliefs are transferred to us from the people around us. These beliefs are either positive or negative and may be hidden and limiting. The classic example of a negative limiting belief is of a baby elephant. When the circus trainer catches the baby elephant, he ties its back leg with a chain to the stake. The baby elephant tries, again and again, to make itself free of the stake, but each time it fails. Later, realizing that all its efforts are in vain, it gives up trying and grows old. As a mature adult elephant, it can now easily pull out the stake, but it had way back, developed the belief that it can't escape from the stake. So, it stays there without trying, for the rest of its life, even though the trainer ties the big elephant merely with a rope.

So, what happens when we believe something. Beliefs decide the boundaries of our understanding, our perception. These numerous beliefs, some positive and some limiting and negative, shape our personality, control and direct our behavior, decide our responses. These beliefs can make you or break you. You become what you believe.

When Shivaji, the great king of Maharashtra, was young, his mother Jijau would tell him the stories from the great epics of Ramayana and Mahabharata. She would tell him the stories about Lord Rama, how he killed Ravana, and the stories of Lord Krishna, and how he killed Kansa and made the people free from the unjust rule of these cruel kings. The young Shivaji was very much fond of listening to the stories of these great heroes of India and when his mother would tell him that he was the heir of these great people. He can also make his people free from the unjust rule of Nizam, Mughals, and Adilshaha, who then used to fight often among each other and never cared for the people's welfare. Her words would ignite and fill his mind with the ideas of doing heroic deeds like Lord Rama, Krishna, and Arjuna. She made him believe that he was there to establish his own rule, own kingdom, unlike his father, who was serving other rulers. As Shivaji had a deep faith and respect towards his mother, he believed sincerely in each word she uttered. And at the age of 14, he took the oath of establishing

Hindavi Swarajya and won his first fort at 16.

When we believe something 100%, our mind gets absolute assurance from within and never thinks anything negative and remains totally positive for that particular thing. And being so positive, as we have seen in the chapter on thinking, we now know the brain starts creating positive images and pictures. Mind with complete faith and belief focuses on results and rewards; thoughts of fear and doubt do not interfere at all. With such an assured mindset and conviction, the mind becomes cool, calm, and with undivided focus, works with 100% concentration, and accomplishes the task successfully. It is as if Julius Caesar said, *'I came, I saw, and I won.'*

Complete belief in ourselves gives us immense power. Such people perform exceptionally well, without getting tired and bored. These people can easily access the inner force and the infinite intelligence.

With such firm belief, the positive images in mind trigger the brain to release the positive chemicals in the blood. The body's homeostasis is maintained; we feel happy, energetic, and the creativity turns on. We focus better, respond better, make better choices, and get better results, ultimately everything goes well. If this cycle persists for a sufficient period, our body gets addicted to these positive chemicals released by the brain. Once this happens, these people find a way to be happy and successful every single day with that positive state of mind. The subconscious mind and body manifest the circumstances, where the brain has to release these chemicals repeatedly.

When we believe something firmly, our brain feels comfortable with the new situation, and the inner resistance for change is reduced totally. So, our body and the mind, accepts the desired change smoothly.

The science of the placebo

It is now well known that nearly one-third of the total medicines available in the pharmaceutical industry are placebos. Placebos are like sugar pills, do nothing. But when they are given, by the authority with a convincing voice, that it will cure the pain, and the patients believe it undoubtedly, and it really cures the pain.

There are numerous evidence and cases where Doctors have witnessed that the placebo has cured the patients and healed the diseases. In one such incident, where a woman was suffering from vomiting and severe nausea, and whose reports revealed her disrupted gastric conditions, on offering a medicine, which actually used to induce nausea, by an authority figure and she was told," this is the most effective medicine and undoubtedly cure your complaints." She indeed believed the medication and the doctor's words, and after some time, she was reported normal, and her gastric tests were also showing the usual pattern. This is precisely why some Doctors become more popular because they use their influence and exercise the power of belief in patients to get them cured. With belief in the medicine and the doctor, the patient's brain starts the biochemical reactions to bring the expected result.

In one such similar incident, when a prisoner was sentenced to death, it was told to him that he would be given the death sentence by the snake bite. At the time of execution, he was blindfolded and was pricked with needles. Assuming that the snake bit him, he indeed died. And when the autopsy was performed, it was found that he was died of the chemicals, similar to snake's venom. This story may be true or may not be, but our brain is indeed capable of doing this.

In India, we hear a very popular story of saint Meerabai, a devotee of Lord Krishna from the province of Rajasthan, in 16 th century. She was married to the Rajput king Bhojraj Sisodiya. But, in her childhood, she had accepted Lord Krishna as her husband and devoted her whole life in devotion and love for her deity. She is a prominent figure in the Bhakti movement in North India. It is said and believed widely that when she was given the milk with poison by her in-laws, who were trying to persecute her, nothing happened. The poison could not do her any harm because she had a firm belief in her God.

In India, as a part of religious tradition, people walk on the burning coals, insert needles in their bodies, beat themselves with razor-sharp blades, and nothing happens to them. It's all because they have faith in it. As we believe, so shall we receive.

I know one such incident, where a woman had a snakebite, few hours before she came to know about it. But it didn't affect her. But the moment she realized it was a snake bite, she died. It's true; people die if they believe.

This belief in our life is the most potent force. Without belief of some kind, positive or negative, we can't move ahead. If we look carefully, every moment of our life is filled with risk. There is a factor of uncertainty in everything, and anything can happen to us at any moment. We don't have control over numerous things. We can hear the news of our beloved ones' demise anytime. We may face an accident, and an earthquake can happen. We may fall on the head and lose our life, or we may not wake up the following day from our sleep. It's all possible. The sun may not rise tomorrow. In fact, we are living a very uncertain life. But, even then, we keep on living, dreaming, keep doing all the desired things, just believing that everything will go well. We just believe unconsciously. This belief makes us live, plan and go ahead. Without this belief, we can't survive. Our beliefs create the world for us.

Whether it be a temple, a church or a mosque, or anything else, all the worshiping places are actually the refueling centers of faith and belief. And the faith or belief in itself is magical. It is the guiding force behind everything.

Everything that exists in our life may be good or bad, is there because we believe it. There are worries, sorrows, problems. All exist because we believe in their existence. Therefore, they are there. If we can believe, everything is well, and life is beautiful, so will it be. If you can believe yourself strong, strong, you will be. The moment we believe it, the brain starts producing the essential chemicals that will make you strong.

The answer to our problem is our beliefs. You have to believe 100%.

You can build new beliefs with powerful affirmations. I will be talking about some efficient ways of forming firm beliefs in forthcoming chapters.

Chapter 6

Perception; the ultimate solution to all problems

We don't see things as they are; we see things as we are...

Anais Nin.

Perception is the word derived from the Latin word **perceptio**, which means gathering or receiving. Perception is different from thinking. It is the interpretation of thoughts and other sensory information. It mainly depends upon the purpose or motive of the observer.

The other factors that influence perception are your level of information, beliefs, and past experiences. In everyday life, we see the world around us and perceive it as the influence of the above factors. And we respond accordingly. But the world doesn't need to be precisely the same as our perception. The real world is always different.

Our perception decides the quality of our life.

There is a famous story in Mahabharata, the Hindu's religious epic. According to Hindu mythology, Lord Krishna, one of the deities, who is considered the eighth incarnation of Lord Vishnu, plays a prominent role in the story of Mahabharata. It is the story of a family, and the family's children were the cousins of Lord Krishna. Pandavas were five brothers, and Kauravas were believed to be 100 in number. Pandavas were very noble and sincere, followed the path of Dharma, and Kauravas were quite the opposite in nature. They were very greedy and proud. Yudhistira was the eldest among the Pandavas, and Duryodhana was Kaurava's eldest brother.

Once in a ceremony, and there were many kings and ministers from different states had also gathered. Lord Krishna called the Yudhistira and asked him to make a round in the pendaal (spectators' area) and find out at least one impious person. Yudhishtira went to look and searched and found that all of those present were pious and had some noble qualities. He returned to Krishna and told him that all the attendees were noble people and no one with bad character.

Then Krishna called Duryodhana and asked him to look for at least one person with a noble character. Duryodhana went and saw the kings and the ministers gathered there and all others. When he started looking at each of them, he could only find their faults and see their bad qualities. He returned to Krishna and said, 'O my Lord, there is not even a single noble person in this crowd. I found everyone with some evil character.

The moral of the story is that it is not what you look at that matters, but it is what you see. Your perception can make a heaven out of hell and the hell out of heaven.

In the darkness, you look at a piece of the rope and perceive it as a snake. This perception of a rope as a snake changes your biochemistry. Your heartbeat goes up, you begin to sweat, and within seconds your body is switched into flight or fight mode. you either try to kill it with whatever you have, or you jump away from there.

Your perception decides your experiences. It also determines your limitations. We know the story of David, the shepherd boy, once went to meet his brothers, who were in the army of Israel and were fighting against the philistines Goliath, the giant, and were very much afraid of him. When David asked his brother," why don't you kill the giant?' his brother answered," can't you see, he is so big to hit." David replied, "No, he is too big to miss," and we know the story, how David killed Goliath with his slingshot. The change in perception changed the result of the battle.

Most of our problems of fear, worries arise due to misperception. Fear is nothing but negative imagination, which comes out due to inadequate perception.

Whatever inside is found outside, whenever you find yourself in anguish or find yourself worried, you will face more circumstances that will make you more worried, so change your perception about the things causing you pain. Our perception can be altered in almost all situations. Always try to be well informed. Or simply change your perspective.

This implies that if you are facing a problem, the real problem is in your perception. And so, perception can literally solve any of your problems.

In the next chapter, I will be telling you some of the most inspiring stories that can really change your perception.

Chapter 7

Character, the foundation for Achieving Greatness

If Wealth is lost, nothing is lost.

If Health is lost, something is lost.

But if Character is lost, everything is lost.

Billy Graham.

When I was in school, I used to read these lines written on the school wall. But I hardly understood the meaning of the last sentence. I had a very vague idea about character. Slowly and gradually, it dawned upon me the meaning of the term, the Strength of Character. By the dictionary meaning, the term character refers to an individual's distinctive mental and moral qualities. These qualities include Honesty, Integrity,

Dedication, Determination, Perseverance, Courage, Patience, and other such attributes together form a good character. There are also qualities like greed, laziness, dishonesty, indiscipline, and other such attributes that create a bad character.

The character has a two-way effect. It affects the people around us as well as on our self. What happens when we compromise with our values when we use shortcuts. Remember when we cheat somebody, tell a lie to our parents, or steal something or try to copy in the exam, we feel weak from within. We get frightened easily, lose our inner strength, lose our peace of mind. And we lose our self-respect though some of us may not realize it at that moment. But the symptoms can be seen clearly, looking at their behavior, which always displays the character. Such people can't think clearly, can't talk with confidence, feel afraid from within. They change their stand quickly.

They lose their stability. People use shortcuts to win, and by doing so, fail in long runs of life.

Every human aspires to achieve something in his life, like success, happiness, health, riches, strong relations, love, respect, and essential things for a fulfilled life. But without a rock-solid character, none of the above stays with us. Talent or ability can take us high, but ultimately it is the character that keeps us flying high.

With a strong character comes the sense of fulfillment, mind being assured, stays calm and confident, self-respect goes up. Body's homeostasis is maintained. The immune system becomes strong. The mind is at rest, thinks positive and clear; creativity turns on, makes the right decisions, gets the right results, and everything goes well. Indeed, Character is the foundation on which huge successful life can be built.

Mark Murphy, the author of Hiring for Attitude, talks about the failure among the new hires. According to him, 89% of the new employees fail due to their attitude, and only 11% fail for the lack of skills. Jeff Keller says, *'Your attitude is your window to the world.'*

If we look at the lives of the great people of past and present, we can notice that it is their character that made them achieve the greatness, took them to that great height. They had or have one or more prominent traits of the good characters, which dominated their personality and influenced the lives of the people around them.

If we look at the life of Mahatma Gandhi, we notice, **truthfulness**, one of his major weapons, in fighting against the British, was the prominent trait of his character. Though he had some other influential qualities, I want to focus on this quality of his character.

When he was a child, he had seen the Drama on the life of great ancient king

Harishchandra, who is the epitome of truth. His life story was full of great ordeals, but he never compromised with truth and his commitment. His story made an indelible impression on the young Gandhi's mind, and since that early age, he was committed to truthfulness and never compromised. He would always think to be like Harishchandra, standing by the truth in all walks of life. He talks about one such incident in his Autobiography.

Once a school inspector had visited his class and asked the students to write few words. One among those words was Kettle, which Gandhi couldn't write. On seeing this, his teacher prompted him to copy from the notebook of another student. But he didn't; in fact, he couldn't understand what the teacher was trying.

The next day, when the teacher called him a fool for not copying the word from others' notebooks, Gandhi felt miserably sorry for the teacher for asking him to copy. He had a firm belief in the truth. Satyagraha was his unique way of fighting against injustice. His commitment to truthfulness made him The Father of the Nation.

If we look at the life of Narendra Modi, India's most influential prime minister, India has ever seen, who once used to sell tea on a railway platform with his father, achieved this greatness because of his quality of **Dedication.** He has been working nearly 19 hours a day, seven days per week, since he was elected as the Prime minister of India, since May 2014, without taking a single holiday, not even on Sundays. He calls himself Pradhan Sevak, which means The Chief Servant of the nation.

Earlier to this, during the 2014 general elections, he made historic campaigning. He addressed more than 5827 rallies, programs, and events, traveled more than 3 lakh kilometers, over the 25 states of India, with a unique vision for each state. Though he traveled far across the country during those days, giving speeches in different cities, he used to return late in the night to his residence in his home state. Then he would personally check all his emails and messages before going to bed, probably by 1:30 or 2 am, and would wake up by 5:30 am, in the morning, every single day. He sleeps for three and half hours only.

His complete dedication with the deepest faith towards the service of Motherland gives him the inner force, and that is the secret of his relentless energy and enthusiasm, with which he has been working unremittingly. He has such a strong Character. Although I am talking about his dedication only, he is a living legend, a perfect example of a man of principles.

The quality of **perseverance** or **persistence** is more effective than the talent in shaping the quality of life and achieving greatness.

"In the confrontation between the stream and the rock, the stream always wins- not through strength but by perseverance." –
H. Jackson Brown

The classic example of perseverance is the invention of the Light Bulb by **Thomas Alva Edison**. He says, "*I have not failed. I have just found 10,000 ways that won't work.*"

And it took him more than ten years to invent the light bulb. In an attempt to use the quality filament for the bulb, he had started his own mining plant to get the quality ore. After ten years of efforts, he still couldn't find the suitable ore for his filament. Edison didn't stop, and he kept going.

Edison says, "*Our greatest weakness lies in giving up. The most certain way to succeed is always to try just one more time.*" He is the epitome of perseverance. This quality of perseverance turned an ordinary hard-of-hearing boy into an extraordinary inventor and made him immortal with his inventions.

This characteristic trait of perseverance of Henry Ford, the founder of Ford company, made him invent the impossible V8 engine with eight cylinders, which revolutionized the car industry. This engine's structural requirement was considered very difficult and was supposed to be impossible to produce. Henry Ford called his engineers and put forth his idea of creating a V8 engine. They knew that it was an impossible task to accomplish. They said, "you are our master, we can't argue with you, but this can't be done.' Ford was very reluctant, he told them that he knew it could be done, and he believed in his men. He asked them to go and build the engine. Six months went by, nothing happened. Eight months went by; still, nothing happened. He just ordered them to keep on trying.

One year passed, nothing could be achieved. The engineers came to report him, and they were very disappointed. But Henry Ford was a man of vision. He said,' Go and built the engine. I know it can be built. And don't come to me till you achieve it.' That left the engineers with no option but to invent it. They pursued it hard, tried every bit, left no stone unturned, and finally, they made it. It happened in 1932. Ford launched the car with a V8 engine at the most affordable price that could run 75 miles per hour. It was all before world war 2. It was an outstanding achievement at that time.

The truest wisdom is a resolute determination. – **Napoleon Bonaparte.**

The level of **Determination** determines the level of success. It is the highest quality that can make anyone successful. The man with such a determined mindset achieves his goal, no matter what comes in between. Irrespective of all odds and pains, irrespective of all the situations and circumstances, he achieves success.

Arunima Sinha is the first female Indian amputee to climb Mount Everest. She was a national volleyball player and wanted to pursue her interest in sports. So, she applied for a job in CISF.

On 12 April 2011, she had boarded a train to Delhi to appear for the exam. On that unfortunate day, her life changed totally; when she resisted the robbers from snatching her chain, she was thrown away from the running train. She felled on the parallel rail track, and the train passed from over her left leg. She became unconscious for a while. She was there, in the middle of the two rail tracks, with all that unbearable pain, shouting for help throughout the night. It was the dark night of her life, trains were passing from both sides, but nobody came there to help her.

The next morning, when she was hospitalized, she got amputated her leg below the knee. The visitors took pity on her. But she wanted to prove herself. Lying on the bed in the hospital, she was thinking of achieving something massive and big. And she decided to climb the world's highest peak, Mount Everest, and wanted to show the world her mettle. After just two days of rest, she started to walk with her prosthetic limb, which showed her strong **determination.**

By March 2012, she started her training without taking a holiday. For her, there was no Sunday, no festival. In the very next year, she began to climb the highest peak in the world. Climbing on Mount Everest with the prosthetic leg was a big challenge. There were some spots, during the trek, where she had no ladders for the support over the wide gaps, there she had to jump over; if she missed it, she would have lost her life.

Arunima faced more difficulties due to her artificial leg. It was very unstable on the ice. She couldn't even care for her wounds in fear of her amputated leg getting frostbite, so she didn't remove the gloves also.

She took 52 days to reach the top of the highest peak. It was on 21 May 2013; She was on top of the world. She was awarded with Padmshree, India's fourth-highest civilian award, for her achievement. Now, after achieving this, she is determined to climb the highest mountains in each continent. She is a perfect example of **determination** and has become an inspiration for the youth.

I can't stop myself from talking about the man with only hand, Karoly Takacs. He was a Hungarian Sergeant. In 1939, he was 28 years old, and by that time, he had won many national and international awards, so he was being considered the strong contender of Gold Medal in shooting for the 1940 Tokyo Olympics.

Then the disaster struck. In a training camp, a grenade exploded in his right hand, his shooting hand, and he lost his hand. All hopes could have gone with the gone hand for anyone, but not for the man of **determination** like Karoly.

With his hand lost, he could have given up his dream of winning a gold medal in the Olympics of 1940. But only after months of treatment in the hospital he focused on what he was left with, his only left hand.

Soon, he began practicing with his left hand. Only after one year he was at National Championship. His friends were delighted to see him there to cheer for them but were surprised when Karoly told them that he was not there to cheer for them but to compete with them. And he won that National Championship.

Now, he was very eager to participate in the Olympics. But due to World War 2, the two consecutive Olympic Games were postponed. But he was determined. And he waited for eight years till the 1948 Olympics to fulfil his dream with the same zeal. He won the Gold medal in shooting not only in the 1948 Olympics but in the 1952 Olympics too. That was the result of his strong, unwavering determination.

I think an ability to **Focus** on the desired thing is one of the most powerful traits of a strong character. I can remember one name very prominently among a few worth mentioning is the name of Sachin Tendulkar. When he was 15 years old, he and his schoolmate Vinod Kambli scored 664 runs while playing in an inter-school competition. It was a record partnership for any wicket in any class of cricket. That partnership opened the doors of their selection in Mumbai team and team India.

Both of them were equally talented, with high potential. But the difference was of **focus**. Soon after their initial success at the international level, Vinod Kambli couldn't carry on the quality of his original game. But Sachin's story is quite different. His success never could shift his focus to anywhere else rather than cricket. Throughout his career of 24 years, he played for the sake of the game itself, purely out of passion. He always considered the game of cricket above everything and more important than anything else. During these 24 years of his career, he had many ups and downs, faced criticism, gone through many bad patches, suffered injuries. But none of these could divert his focus from the game of cricket. He has been humble and down to Earth. It is said that he practiced every single day, wherever he would go. He is the only batsman who made centuries of centuries and the only sportsman who has been conferred upon the title of BharatRatna, the highest civilian award. The cricketing world calls him The God of Cricket.

Finally, it is the **hard work** that pays for sure. The story of the highest Gold medal winner in the Olympics, Michael Phelps, who is considered the most outstanding athlete ever, who has won 28 Olympic medals out of which 23 are gold, and the number is greater than the total medals achieved by 161 countries together.

He attributes his success to his coach Bowman, who recognized Phelps's potential and encouraged him to push hard. Phelps would swim for 80000 meters per week. It is almost 50 miles. He dominated the swimming world for two decades across five Olympics. His best performance was in the 2008 Beijing Olympics, where he won all the eight gold medals in all the categories of swimming, butterfly, freestyle, and Medlock. At the time of his seventh victory over a Serbian Milorad Cavic, he won by one-hundredth of a second. It is said that, he could do that because, when he was injured, a small bone of his right wrist was broken before the Olympics, and he was unable to use his hands more; that time, he had focused and practiced more on back kicking. He talks about his hard work in his book**, No Limits**: "For five years, from 1998 to 2003, we did not believe in days off. I had one because of a snowstorm, two more due to the removal of wisdom teeth. Christmas?

See you at the pool. Thanksgiving? Pool. Birthdays? Pool. Sponsor obligations? Work them out around practice time." Hard work really paid him.

Though I have focused on only one quality from the above great people's personalities, in the true sense, they have many other attributes that helped them in moulding their lives and achieving greatness. The characteristic traits I mentioned are the few among those important qualities, which make a person reach great heights. Each of the above attributes has immense value.

Being truthful gives you enormous strength from within. Truth being eternal is omnipresent, so it is said, **Satyamev Jayate**. Truth always triumphs.

Dedication is the state when you have it, your mind, heart, and body are totally immersed, and you have unwavering faith. That gives you access to your inner force, and you become unstoppable.

Determined people are those People who have complete self-control and complete control over their thoughts and emotions. They can achieve anything.

And people who can focus use their minds' secret power because whatever you focus on, the mind starts getting attracted to it. And once you start taking an interest in something, the hardship in pursuing it becomes a pleasure. And finally, it is the hard work that accomplishes the goals.

Patience, courage, responsibility, empathy, compassion, and integrity are some other traits of a strong character. People with these qualities can do anything, can exercise their highest potential, exhibit their immense power. So, the strong character builds their destiny. And that is why: if the character is lost, everything is lost.

It is said that character is the result of our habits. So, in our next chapter, we will check in the science behind the habits.

Chapter 8

The Science of Habit

We are what we repeatedly do.

Aristotle.

Habits are automated, repeated actions. They are under our subconscious control. The Southern California University research says 40 to 45 % of our behavior is the result of our habits. We perform our habitual actions without getting aware of them, without our conscious efforts. This happens because of our brain. Though the size of the human brain is only 2% of our body, it consumes 20% of the total energy and oxygen supply. Hence, our brain always calculates the amount of energy needed for doing a particular thing. It is always up to saving energy. So, when the action is repeated, those specific synapses become stronger and stronger, and the action gets performed automatically to save time and energy. Like, when we drive a car or bike, we do not change the gears consciously. But at the first time of driving a car or learning anything new, the brain needs to focus a lot and put a lot of energy in use. Once it becomes easy, it becomes a part of a habit. And the subconscious mind takes control of it. It happens because our conscious mind can focus upon 2 or 3 crucial actions at a time. But the subconscious mind has immense power.

Unfortunately, our brain can't differentiate between good and bad habits.

Naturally, when teenage starts, our brain also passes through the stage called Synoptic pruning. This stage is also known as Use it or Lose it.

What happens is, the brain starts eliminating the unnecessary synapsis, and only those synapses get stronger, which are in use. It occurs because the brain is preparing itself to function at a more complex level. That's why teenage is a crucial period for habit formation, behavior consolidation, and molding personality. That's why it has been found that 80% of smokers got habituated before the age of 18.

We create habits, and habits create us back. Our habits become our character, and we know our character is our destiny.

Brian Tracy says, "*Form good habits and make them your master, although good habits are hard to form but easy to live with and bad habits are easy to form but hard to live with.*"

Today we can learn new habits effortlessly, and we can eliminate the bad ones too.

Let's understand the science of habit. Any repeated action that turns into habit passes through cycle of 3 R stages, as Charles Duhigg talks about it.

The first R is **Reminder**. It may be a place, time, or particular thing that triggers a specific action: the second R, **Routine**. And when the action is taken, we get the **Reward** (3rd R) of joy, satisfaction, or we feel good. It happens because when we perform the action, our brain releases dopamine. Dopamine makes us happy, feel good. Our brain registers this reminder, cue as significant, which results in making us feel good. So, whenever we find the reminder or the signal, we are tempted to take action, respond unconsciously, and get the reward of dopamine. This dopamine is a chemical and is like a drug, and the body gets habituated to it. The body demands this chemical, and we are forced to perform the action, again and again, irrespective of its significance.

But today, we can change our bad habits, and we can form new desired habits. We can use NLP, visualization, and affirmations to get rid of our bad habits. And to develop new habits, James Clear, in his book 'The Atomic Habits' talks about the habit stacking method. It works wonderfully. Whatever the new habit you want to adopt, just look at your present habits and, considering the time, and location associate the new desired habit or action with the past one. We have to repeat the new action immediately after the old routine, every single day, till it becomes automatic.

I want to tell you about a bad habit that is considered the number one reason for failure and how we can get rid of it and also about a habit that can make you achieve any success.

First, we will talk about bad habit. We will discuss the practice of **procrastination**, which is the number one cause of failure.

Most of us fall prey to this bad habit at some point in time and suffer a heavy loss due to procrastination. We will go deep into it. In reality, procrastination is the symptom, not the real cause of our failure. If we look keenly, we can understand that people procrastinate when they are overwhelmed, when they do not have a clear vision or when they do not have a specific purpose. Mind being confused tends to avoid to confront.

Secondly, when we set something huge to achieve, we procrastinate because of our brain's natural autopilot functioning. Naturally, our brain's primary role is to keep us safe and avoid pain. And it likes comfort. When we decide to go for something big, which is far out of our comfort zone, our brain certainly avoids it by procrastinating. It gives several noble reasons for avoiding. Being the lover of comfort, it always seeks instant gratification.

We have already seen that everything that matters for our brain is to be in the present tense. It responds in the present, so it tries to seek gratification now. So, it makes you indulge in seeking pleasures in those things that are readily available.

The third reason is that when we are afraid of facing something, or when we feel stressed doing something, that causes our brain to release Cortisol, the stress hormone, as we have seen, creates the fight or flight response in our body. As we are already afraid of doing it, feeling stressed, the brain usually avoids it by making us fly from the situation, and we keep on procrastinating. However, even if you keep on procrastinating, the problem keeps getting worse, and the pressure goes on building.

To overcome this habit of procrastination, you need to make yourself more aware of the situation, scrutinize the pros and cons, consider all the consequences. You should exploit the nature of the human brain, which loves comfort. So, you should divide the big task into small measurable goals, put them just outside of your comfort zone. So that brain will not tend to procrastinate. You can also use visualization added with emotions about the desired future and make your brain more comfortable with it; that way, our subconscious mind works on it and quickly brings those things into reality. When you focus more on the rewards and the benefits of achieving the big task, you feel motivated enough to take the necessary actions, and once you start taking action, everything falls in its place.

The second most important habit I want to talk about is the habit of self-discipline. Everything is possible with this habit, and nothing works without self-discipline. **Elbert Hubbard** defines this habit as" ***Self-discipline*** *is the ability to make yourself do what you should do, when you* *should do it, whether you feel like it or not."* When we do whatever is needed to be done, irrespective of our mood, feelings, and likings, it builds our inner strength, gives us self-control, and our self-esteem goes high. We become more confident. We can set any goals and achieve them.

Quite the opposite to this, when you make a new resolution, particularly on the eve of the new year, and you follow it religiously in the beginning, but soon after a week or two, when you start giving excuses and start skipping the routine, or act against the resolution, with every such act you begin losing your self-control, start losing your self-esteem, and it starts draining your inner strength. Doing anything against your determination makes you week and fickle. Skipping necessary action at times, failing to stick to the resolution, never makes our mind strong. And so, at the time of a big game, we invariably fail to adhere to the important resolution.

To make our life successful, we have to win every day, make the most out of each day. To do this, we need to be consistent every day, and to be consistent every day, we need to have a consistent morning every single day. So, developing morning habits is the real key to have a successful life.

These morning habits should include meditation, expressing gratitude, using strong affirmations, reading self-help books, and exercising. Make a habit of setting your mind and body in the right tone every single morning.

I will reveal a crucial secret of forming new habits permanently, in the next chapter on self-image.

Chapter 9

Self-image, the man in the mirror

People walk through life trying to know others, and the whole life passes without knowing themselves.   Shirish.

Self-image is the concept of your personality; you believe you are in your mind.

The concept of self-image is first discovered by dr. Maxwell Maltz. He was a plastic surgeon. He made this discovery when he found that some of his patients behaved differently even after removing the scars from their faces. After the surgery, those with a healthy self-image became normal and were as confident as they were earlier, but those, who had low self-image, even after the surgery, when they were looking well, didn't feel well. He also noticed few patients who didn't feel low though having scars on the face. The mark on their face didn't affect their confidence. That made him realize and discover the concept of self-image.

Unfortunately, your self-image is not formed by you. It is the outcome of the experiences you get in your early life. The opinions of your parents, friends, relatives, and neighbors about you, and your interpretation of all these, together form your self-image, which works as the basis of all your responses to the external world. It is your spectacle through which you look at the world.

There are three different aspects of your self-image. The one which you believe, you are. The second, the people around you, think as you are, and the third, it is the real you, as you are, it is quite different from the first two.

Our mind has a unique habit of using our past experiences as references for every single situation. These past experiences and our perception of them determine our self-image, which decides how we respond. If the memories of these experiences are happy, healthy, we have an adequate healthy self-Image. If these experiences are bad, unpleasant, our self-image becomes low and inadequate, leading us to underperform and lead a miserable life.

So, we should remember the past successes and remind ourselves of them time and again. That will help us, choosing suitable options, feeling better from within, responding well. And with enough of this practice, we build our healthy self-image, and so our self-image is nothing but our own experience of ourselves.

Why is Self-image so critical?

Self-image is the mirror, which reflects your inner self, out in the external world. There is a science. whatever is inside is reflected outside. We can change our self-image at any given point in time, but most of us are unaware of it.

Till the age of seven, as a child, our brain passes through a programming state, where our brain remains in the theta waves. It receives the information from the surroundings and gets programmed without scrutinizing its significance. In this period, the opinions and the remarks heard about our self are accepted as true and are turned into beliefs.

Once our opinions get confirmed, we start behaving, reacting, expecting in the same way that matches our self-perceived personality. When we start acting, responding in the same manner, our neural pathways get confirmed and become stronger. The confirmed neural pathways represent particular behavior or some specific thoughts or beliefs. As the thoughts and the beliefs, the brain releases certain chemicals, and our body gets addicted to those chemicals. They, in turn, create specific emotions, and the emotions are nothing but energy in motion. They produce vibrations of a particular frequency. As our vibes attract our tribes, the universe reciprocates with similar vibrations. We receive the experiences as we set our vibrations, which are basically the result of our thoughts and beliefs. They are there because of our programming, and due to this programming, we have built our self-image. So, the external world is the reflection of the inner world.

As long as we are carrying the wrong self-image, we will keep facing the same circumstances. We feel low from within and inadequate, which leads to resentment, underperformance, fear, and doubt, all leading to an unhappy life.

We all know the story of an ugly duckling. Once, the duck was waiting to hatch her eggs. One among the eggs was bigger and brighter. When all the eggs hatched, all the baby ducklings started making noise with the sound of quack-quack, except the one, which had come out of that big egg, with grey feathers and a different beak, was looking ugly.

All the ducklings started teasing the ugly duckling. The poor ugly duckling felt very sorry because it couldn't make the sound like others, couldn't swim like other siblings, and saw herself as different and ugly. So, she was very nervous.

The days and months passed; all the siblings grew big. The ugly duckling had also grown with beautiful white feathers and a beautiful beak. But it was very unhappy as the other ducks had been teasing her for her uniqueness.

One day, the folk of swan came into their pond. They were all with beautiful white feathers and beautiful beaks, exactly the same as the ugly duckling. Looking at them and looking at her own reflection in the water, the ugly duckling realized her true self and flew away with the flock of swans and became happy.

Her realization of her true self turned her entire miserable life into the happy one.

The simplest way of building a healthy self-image is to develop good habits. These habits will give you good experiences and shreds of evidence with which you can believe in your self-worth and sufficient of these experiences will build your healthy self-image. And the opposite of this can also work if you can hold the relevant new self-image in your mind; forming new habits become pretty more effortless.

You can use affirmations to build your self-image. The quality of your self-talk decides your self-worth. You can change your beliefs about yourself. You can focus on your future, visualize it, and considering how you want to become the type of person you will be. You can start living like it right from this moment.

We now know that we can fool our brains, and it can't differentiate between reality and imagination. We also know that our brain loves familiarity. When your body and brain get habituated with your future self, your self-image becomes consolidated. Besides this, the law of attraction works and manifests your future.

The second most important thing to build a strong self-image is to accept responsibility. If you can understand and realize that you are alone responsible for your present circumstances, that may be your health, finances, career, and your relations, anything that happened with you. You are responsible for it because your responses are always in your hands. The moment you accept this responsibility and stop blaming and complaining, your self-image goes high.

The third thing you can do to improve your self-image is to avoid the company of negative people, who always indulge in complaining, blaming, comparing, and criticizing. Instead, find the people who value your opinions. They are like-minded people. During the conversation, when your views are accepted and heard with due respect, your brain increases the level of dopamine and serotonin, which makes you feel more empowered and improves your self-image.

Goal setting also helps in building self-image. Well, this is an indispensable topic for achieving greatness. So, we will discuss it's all key issues in the next chapter.

Chapter 10

Goal setting; setting the sail

Nature and nurture have made each one of us unique. From that perspective, everybody has an inimitable purpose in life. We need to figure it out.

With such remarkable discoveries and inventions, man can achieve anything in today's world. The Internet has made this easier. But at the same time, life has become faster, more complex, prone to more distractions.

Today, like never before, more avenues are wide open. So, it is quite natural to get distracted and lead life according to the circumstances. But without purpose, life will be like a boat without sail, which keeps changing the direction as per the direction of the wind. And the sailor will never know where the boat will land. As the philosopher **Seneca** said, "*If one does not know to which port one is sailing, no wind is favorable.*"

Our life is like fertile land, and something must grow out of it. If You don't choose what to grow in your land, weeds will grow for sure.

Zig Ziglar said,*" your life is the result of your choices you have made. If you don't like your life, start making better choices."*

If you don't know where you are heading, how your life will be after five years, ten years, then how Can you make better choices and make the right decisions?

Irrespective of any circumstances, we can design our future, and it is equally possible and has been proved that we can bring it into reality.

I have been focusing more on science, particularly neuroscience, to make you realize that whatever I am talking about is possible and is fool proof.

Our brain has an autopilot goal-seeking mechanism. It is called **Reticular Activating system**. RAS is the cluster of cells located at the base of the brain stem. It processes all the sensory information and filters it, and brings forth only the most appropriate information before you for that moment. The RAS is aware of what you are paying attention to at this very moment, and hence it chooses to focus only on the information related to it. It means that your RAS is doing its job at any given point in time, providing you with the necessary information, but you have not given it the right job if you have not decided what exactly you want in your life. The moment you determine your future, your RAS is ready to help you reach there. You might have noticed that when you decide to do something, you immediately begin to see the relevant things everywhere. These relevant things, which are considered significant now, were there earlier too, but you didn't notice, and now are brought to your attention automatically.

In fact, our brain is malleable, and when we set goals to achieve, our brain is restructured, called Neuroplasticity, to make us perform better and achieve the goals. When you set high and challenging goals, it is found that your brain performs better. You get more motivated when you have an emotional attachment to your destination. And when you perceive your goals achievable, as Rex Wright, a psychologist at the University of North Texas, says, your Systolic Blood Pressure rises, which increases your readiness to take action.

Suppose you perceive your goals that are too big and very distant. In that case, your Medial prefrontal cortex, the part of the brain, which evaluates things, assesses the situations, and makes the decisions, lowers its activation. That is why you lose interest in pursuing goals. To keep yourself pursuing the big goals, break them into small achievable parts.

When you break your big goals into small parts and celebrate after accomplishing each segment, you remain motivated. This happens because, in our brain, there is a small part called **Nucleus Accumbens**, which is responsible for reinforcing rewarding stimuli. That keeps you motivated enough to take action, to get rewarded again.

In short, your brain has everything that can achieve your goal. It is up to you whether you want it or not.

I want to conclude this chapter with the story of Florence Chadwick, an American swimmer and the first woman who swam the English Channel in both directions, setting a record time. She was known for her long-distance open swimming.

In 1952, she decided to swim 26 miles from Catalina Island to California. She swam for 15 hours. The atmosphere was very chilly, and the fog was thicker. She could see only the fog. She lost her hopes and decided to quit. When she boarded the boat, she realized the seashore was only a half-mile away.

The following day, talking to the news reporter, she said, **'If had I seen the seashore, I would have reached it.'**

Only after two months, she started again, swimming from Catalina Island to California seashore. This time also, she couldn't see anything except fog but kept on going because she had her clear goal, the picture of seashore in her mind. And she made it.

If you can see your designed future clearly, you can achieve it definitely.

Goals are like the pole stars; always help to choose the direction. No matter what, you can reach there if you have fixed goals and only if you take action.

We will discuss this topic of great magnitude in our next chapter. I believe this one chapter on action has everything that will make you achieve greatness.

Chapter 11

Action -The only key to success

Apart from all the chapters we discussed earlier, I am purposefully putting this chapter after the goal-setting. However, we all know actions are inevitable after powerful thoughts and affirmations. But it is also evident that people tend to keep thinking and planning as if they have been caught in analysis and paralysis syndrome. They never take the essential step of taking action.

Why I value this one chapter above all the remaining because taking action on your desired goal in the direction of your aspirations and dreams brings all the necessary things to you. With consistent actions every day, even a tiny step towards your goal removes all the stress, lethargy and fills you with Endorphin. This happy drug keeps you energetic and motivated. When you take consistent daily actions, the consistency breeds into developing habits. When you have enough experience of a series of successful activities and positive results, it builds your positive self-identity. You have new beliefs developed in alignment with your goals. Everything seems possible by just making a small effort every day. You stay in a positive state of mind, become more optimistic, and pessimistic thoughts cannot drain your energy. Achieving success becomes as easy.

There may be moments when you feel like not doing anything. Mind being the servant of habits, as the brain prefers convenience, tends to adopt the familiar path. The human brain tends to do those things repeatedly, which pleases it. As the law of inertia and the rule of momentum suggest, when you keep yourself in motion by taking action every day, you are naturally inclined to keep it moving unless and until you break your routine.

Taking action is the only antidote against all the negative thoughts of fear and self-doubt. Action is the only secret behind staying positive. People try to be perfect all the time, but this perfectionism is a kind of syndrome. Imperfect daily actions take you towards achieving excellence.

Positive thinking, using powerful affirmations, believing firmly, having a solid character, and building a healthy, successful self-image any of these or all together won't work if you don't take action every single day.

People say direction is more important than speed. I would suggest speed in the right direction will change your game and let you achieve your ultimate goal without delay. Sometimes it is also possible that you may lose your direction or lose your pace. It's ok and entirely natural. But giving up the efforts and not moving ahead is against nature. If you look at nature, you will find everything is moving. Even the most stationary objects, which seem to be immovable, are in a state of constant motion. In fact, the universe loves motion, movement, and action is the key to be aligned with this ever-changing universe.

Sometimes it may happen that even after your dedicated efforts, you find yourself stuck, not making any progress. It's like a scrap day. Don't worry. Keep on moving with the scrap, and within some time, you will find yourself regaining your momentum. As Robin Sharma says," Change is hard in the beginning, messy in the middle, and gorgeous in the end."

There is a famous saying in Sanskrit. It is ***Uddyamen hi siddhanti Karyani,nach manorathe.Nahi pravishyanti suptasya sinhasy***

mukhe mruga means every work is accomplished by taking actions only and never by just thinking and wishing as how a prey never enters into the mouth of a sleeping lion, though the king of the jungle.

In Bhagavad-Gita, the sacred book of Hindu, there is a very popular verse ***Karmanyevadhikarste ma faleshu kadachan***. It means you consider the actions only, not their results, as you have authority over the action only and do not have control over the results. And if you take right actions, the right result is inevitable.

In the **Holy Bible**, in the New Testament, in the chapter of Mathew's gospel, we find this verse *"knock, and it shall be opened unto you."*

Only wishing, believing, praying won't work unless you do something on it. It is also well said that **'God helps those who help themselves.'**

We know Newton's third law that for every action, there is an equal and opposite reaction. If you take better steps, you will have better results. As you sow, so shall you reap.

The law of karma states that it is the action that governs the whole thing. It suggests that God doesn't give you fruits, but your actions do. Your present life is the result of your past deeds, and your current actions will determine your future.

When you take action every single day, you become unstoppable, and reaching a goal becomes inevitable. And when your actions match with words you speak and thoughts in your mind, you do wonders.

So, **JUST DO IT**...take action every day...Every single day...Remember, the world belongs to the people who take action.

Chapter 12

Time; the principal asset for achieving greatness

If you can fill the unforgiving minute,
With sixty seconds' worth of distance run,
Yours is the Earth and everything that's in it,
And—which is more—you'll be a Man, my son!

Rudyard Kipling

Time is the only valuable asset that each of us has in equal quantity, irrespective of our current status. It is the same for the poor and rich.

For me, time is above all assets. It is above health, above wealth. We can regain our health and wealth, but we can't retrieve the time lost at any cost.

Time is life. If we waste our time, we will be wasting our life. If you value your time, time will make you valuable.

Once a professor wanted to teach something significant to his students. He took a big glass jar, a water bottle, a bag of sand, some pebbles, and few rocks. He poured the water into the jar and fill it completely. Then he filled it with the sand. When he was adding the sand, the water started spilling over. Then he started filling the pebbles, and he could hardly put few stones in the jar, as there was very little space left. Then he picked up the rocks to put in, but he could not put a single rock in it since the jar was already full.

Then he took another jar. But this time, he reversed the entire sequence. First, he put some rocks, and then he added some pebbles to it. They fit well in the spaces between the rocks. He then filled the jar with the sand. The sand occupied the gaps between the rocks and pebbles. Finally, he poured the water and waited till it gets soaked in the sand. Now the entire jar was full.

Few of the students could understand what the professor was about to bring up to them. He then turned to his students and said,' If you fill your jar of life with only trivial things, here water and sand, you will be left with very little time (space) to do big tasks, pursuing your goals. So, prioritize, do the essential things first, minor issues will automatically fall into their place.

When everything is ok, you have no health issues, no financial problems, no significant family problems, realize that this is the best time for you to prepare for your future. We never know the uncertainties in the future. So, invest your time.

The value of time is immense. But only those who achieved greatness know it. If you look at Michael Phelps, who won his seventh gold medal, in 2008, Beijing Olympic, by **the margin of one-hundredth of a second,** you probably will never question the value of time.

When Mark Zuckerberg, the CEO of Facebook, once asked why he wears the same grey-colored T-shirt every day. He gave a very grave answer. He said that he felt lucky to have the opportunity to serve more than a billion people and didn't want to waste his time over making such petty decisions like what to wear, and so wasting time he thinks is not doing his job.

If we consider the average life span of people worldwide as 75 years, we spend nearly 30% of the time sleeping, which is approximately 25 years of our life in bed. If we further calculate the possible time we spend on each routine task, like for eating we spend nearly four years of our life, and keep excluding these times, we will be left with only ten years to do something worthwhile, in our entire stay on this planet.

To put the long story short, I would like you to know that God has given this greatest asset of time equally to each one of us. It is up to you, what you do with that.

To utilize the time to its fullest, we must know the nature of life. I want to tell you some of the most substantial facts about life in the next chapter.

Chapter 13

Knowing the facts of life, essential for achieving greatness

The Story of my brother

Ours was a middle-class family. We were seventeen members, living together, all under one roof, and my father was the only earning hand. He was a teacher in a govt school.

We were three brothers, Nitin Being the eldest and me the youngest. He was six years older than me. But that age difference was never an issue.

My father had made us call each other by the names since our childhood. Calling the elder brother by name was a radical move at that time. My relatives, neighbors would always wonder and object to me for calling my elder brother by his name. They would expect me to call him DADA or ANNA (words for calling elder brother with due respect). We were brought up more like friends. We could chat for hours, on any topic, without hesitation, without any restriction on sharing the secrets between us. When we talk or discuss, we often laugh a lot. Whatever the subject might be, no matter how serious it might be, the discussion would mostly turn out with a positive outcome. A feeling would always be there that our conversation should never stop. There was always joy in being together. That pleasure of living together, eating together, watching the television together, particularly on vacations holidays, watching cricket matches and movies, commenting and cutting jokes, were the happiest moments in my life.

There was a very high-level intimacy and liking for each other. So, the absolute pleasure was the pleasure of being together. Going on a trip together would always add more happiness and joy to our life. And I was surprised when I came to know that each of his friends had felt the same feeling of intimacy while being with Nitin.

He was really a Gem, Noble by nature, and would always run to help others. He was a perfect example of an ideal friend. He was very optimistic by nature.

When I was in primary school, he was in college. He used to play cricket and was the opening batsman of his team. It was a kind of delight, watching his batting. He was very much fond of music. He used to bring different musical instruments at home and play on them. He also loved cooking. The aroma of biryani, he would make, still lingers in my mind. Above all, he had great interest and taste in Plays and dramas.

Then life took over; he got a job and got married. I, too, got a job and got married after few years.

Due to some unavoidable circumstances, we had to stay in different places. Though we were busy in our lives, we used to celebrate the festivals together, in our home town. Particularly in Diwali vacations, when we all brothers and uncle and their families and kids meet, It was indeed a fest, and there were all celebrations. The one among all, the star attraction of the Diwali, was, taking a bath, all together, early in the morning, in the yard, sitting all together on the Mancha(cot), all screaming and shouting for water. Since the ladies would pour water with the jugs on all, sometimes the water would be too hot, or some may not get the water; those who sit in the front row would get more water. This bathing ceremony would last for half an hour but would fill all of us with joy and happiness, which would last for the rest of the year.

Since we were busy with our lives and there were only a few occasions when we could come and live together. We were thinking about it seriously. Therefore, we started our institutional school at our native place. The motive behind starting the school was to get that liberty and opportunity to work and live together. Once school started, we used to meet every Saturday evening and discuss all family and school issues. He had a strong wish to establish our school building and our family residence on our farm, which is on the outskirts of our native town. Sitting in the field, we had spent hours together, talking about our future, about the school, the construction of the school building, our house, and the future of our family.

But the day came. It was on the 30 March 2019, early in the morning at 2 am; I received a call from his wife that he had severe pain in his chest and they were taking him to hospitalize at district place 70 kilometers from his residence. I left home immediately and reached there by 5 am. During that journey, there wasn't a single negative thought in my mind. All that my mind was thinking of hospitalizing him and the possible days it would take to recover. Because, during the journey, I was constantly making the calls and asking the updates. I had been told that his pulse was showing on the movement.

The moment I reached there, in the hospital, in a ward, he was lying on the bed, motionless, as if he was sleeping. Everybody was crying. The Doctor had declared him brought dead. It was all unexpected, unbelievable, and unacceptable. My conscience, mind, heart, and brain were all in no way accepting the truth that happened with my brother. I was trying to wake him up, again and again. I went to Doctor to talk, but he made me realize that it was too late. Nothing could be done, and my brother had gone far away and forever from me.

The very day, by 4 pm, we performed his last ceremony and it all ended in the matter of within 24 hours. Our life had changed entirely in a single day. It was like a nightmare, completely unbelievable.

At the time of his last ceremony, I wept like a child, all frustrated, completely sank in grief, and terribly disappointed. Nothing on the Earth could make me and my heart stop from crying.

It was my first close encounter with death. My mind was constantly thinking of my brother's death. What exactly had happened with him? Where exactly, he might have gone? Why did he leave the game halfway? He had hardly started driving his dream car, which he had bought just three months before he passed away. The day before his death, he was all playing on the synthesizer (musical instrument), full of life, hopes and dreams, and tons of love for his family and friends. How could he go, leaving behind all this and his lovely two kids?

For the next three months, I felt as if he had gone somewhere else, to some unknown place, and would come back any time. But the bitter truth is that he never came to see me and talked with me.

It slowly dawned upon me that each one of us has to leave this place one day, leaving everything behind that is dear to us. I could feel that whatever I am enjoying, possessing at my home, all the luxuries, all the appliances, my family and friends are with me for some more years. I really do not have them forever.

Then why is this system like this? Why people strive throughout life to achieve these things and leave behind everything? Something is wrong, but sure. What is that?

What is death at all? Is everything so meaningless? Such impermanence?

When Goutam Buddha went outside the palace for the first time, completely unaware of the sufferings of life, he saw an older man for the first time. He was told that everybody grows old and becomes weak. Then he met a seek person suffering from a disease. His charioteer Channa said to him that everyone is prone to diseases and has to bear the pain. The two sights had troubled him deeply when he encountered a dead body being carried for the funeral. He was made realize that death is an inevitable fate that befalls everyone.

He was utterly disturbed by the sights, realized the impermanence of life, left his palace and the family, and went into the forest searching for the truth.

Shakespeare also called this life a stage, and all the men and women being the players, and each one has his fixed entrance and exit.

In short, we must never forget the quality of impermanence of this life.

The nature of the universe

Now, the second fact which the achievers of greatness must keep in mind is the nature of the universe. If we look around and consider the size of our milky way Galaxy, consisting of nearly 100 billion stars and the galaxy's length is estimated to take approximately 100,000 years to travel with the speed of light (300000kms/sec). Then there are billions of such galaxies in the universe. The estimated diameter of this universe is 100 billion light-years.

I hope the reader of this book knows what's the light-year? It is the distance traveled by the beam of light in one whole year with a speed of 300000 km per sec. If we decide to put the diameter of the universe in numbers, it would be like this 300000*60*60*24*365*1000000000000 =9460800000000000000000000 Kms. It's just speculation. Nobody knows the exact length. Besides this, scientists have no idea about the number of dimensions of the universe, and they also predict the existence of multiple universes. And man has succeeded somehow in reaching up to Mars so far, which is in our solar system itself. Beyond the solar system, there are 100 billion stars in our galaxy, and beyond our galaxy, there are 100 billion galaxies in the universe.

It's great to explore the universe and reach on the planets, but to know the truth, if we condition ourselves to examine the whole of the universe first and then come to some conclusion, it would be ridiculous. It would be like an ant one trying to explore the whole Earth. However, the Earth has fixed boundaries.

Being human, associating ourselves with this finite body, is next to impossible to see and explore the whole universe with our limitations. But if we can look inside ourselves and know that we are connected with this entire universe, with something inside us, at the fundamental level. Then there will be a possibility that we will understand this universe better.

So, what is that inside us?

Quantum physics says that at the fundamental level, everything is energy. The foundation of this universe is not physical at all. The smallest particles like electrons, muons, tauons, quarks, and gluons are all made of energy, have no physical structure, and are entirely illusory. Moreover, there is no difference between living and non-living things at this level. The smallest particle is found in the wave and particle form at the same time. It all depends on the experiment and the intention of the observer. This wave-particle duality raised questions on the objectivity of science. The observer effect undermined the basic assumption of science about the existence of an objective world. So, in quantum physics, the approach towards reality is that of probabilities.

This happens because of the problem of Epistemology. Epistemology studies the nature of knowledge. At the fundamental level where everything is energy, where the observer, the observed, and the observation are one, or, where the knower, the known, and the knowledge is one, where there is no difference between these, how one is going to describe it, going to put it in words. But the truth is, we are, the ultimate I, that something, which is connected with this infinite universe at that fundamental level, which is within us, is right now, at this very moment and all the time, is always beyond the expression in words. In fact, it is a matter to be experienced, and can't be described, defined, and can't be put in words. And to experience it, we must look inside ourselves.

What our scientists are trying to find out, the true nature of the ultimate form of the fundamental particle; they are actually trying to study it in this external world, outside of themselves, in the laboratory, under the electron microscope. That's why the truth is keeping them eluding.

Einstein said, ***"Reality is merely an illusion, although a very persistent one."*** It will be wise if we remember this.

Limitless knowledge

Humanity is witnessing the fourth revolution—the revolution of information technology. We are living in the information age. In the last thirty years, we have witnessed a massive explosion of information. The information on any given topic is getting doubled every four months.

Suppose we look at the YouTube statics, where nearly 500 hundred hours of videos are being uploaded every single minute, from all across the globe. If we calculate the total hours of videos being uploaded on YouTube per day, we find 720000 hours of videos uploaded every day. This means if someone decides to watch all the videos uploaded in a single day, he will have to keep watching those videos day and night, every day, 24 hours for the next eight years. And with this calculation, we will need more than 240 years to watch all the videos being uploaded in a single month. However, we are talking about the only YouTube here. There are many more such platforms.

To look at this issue differently, if we look at the knowledge, we can see it is related to time and space. As we know, these two parameters are limitless. There is no beginning and end to time and space. Therefore, knowledge is also endless. Though knowing is everything, and knowledge liberates, we are humans with limited resources and time and can't seek the entire empirical knowledge. We can't comprehend precisely how this universe came into existence, how human life evolved on this planet, and will never know the factual history of the world. We have to depend on logical speculations only.

Why people behave like blinds?

1.Your purpose decides your perception. As we have seen, your perception determines your response. It is the result of your beliefs, self-image and depends on the level of your information. Hence, perceptions of life vary from person to person. As your perception is, so is your life.

2. People have programmed sub-conscious minds. Till the age of seven, all of us get programmed from our surroundings. Our nature and nurture have made us unique. So, each one of us has a unique personality. We are running our programs throughout our lives though we haven't chosen them. Our subconscious mind and the surroundings make us think and behave as per our programming.

3. People usually don't think. They do not think about the futurity of what they do. They are always after instant gratification, more concerned with the immediate future. Even though some may think about few steps ahead, but what I want is to think 100X or sometimes 1000X. We have been habituated to think in terms of hours, days, and months. Let's assume you alone have a lifespan of 1000 years. Then you will see, most of the problems, that your family members, friends are facing like the issues of

job, family problems, financial problems, and problems with government and thinking these problems as gigantic are really very small and momentary. In fact, ridiculous. You will see the great things like nations, dynasties, industries, universities rising and falling. You will understand the futurity of everything. You will realize that everything is impermanence.

Here some may think it impractical, but I am talking about the facts of life.

Balance is the key.

We have seen that the universe is infinite, the knowledge is endless, and the knowledge liberates us from ignorance, and knowing is itself gaining everything.

But being humans, we don't do everything for knowing but to experience. To live is to experience, and our life is meant to live.

It is but evident that the experiences that life gives us are very vast. There are innumerable fields to be experienced. With limited resources and limited lifespan, we need to choose the kind of experiences we want in our life. We need to pick our field, our zone of expertise.

To have the totality of experiences and feel the wholeness of life within the timeframe of our lifespan, we need to think of balance. Balance among all the areas of our life. With balance comes the sense of fulfillment.

Your pursuit of good physical health, passionate career, strong relations, financial status, social recognition, enjoying creativity or self-expression, sound emotional and mental health, and your spiritual life should all be in balance. Everything should be in the right proportion, not less, not more. **Extreme of anything** or absence of anything creates an imbalance. The effect of that imbalance can be seen clearly on the overall health of a person. Your rock-solid character lays the foundation for maintaining that balance.

These all areas are like the spokes of a wheel. All essential for smooth running. If we remove or cut, or extend anyone spoke, the wheel of your life will crumble.

However, a perfect balance is quite impossible.

Moreover, it's a lifelong process. Continuous change is the rule of this nature. We need to keep maintaining the balance continuously like a duck, which apparently looks calm while swimming, but it keeps moving its legs continuously under the water.

There is one more problem with maintaining the balance. There is a threat of ending up in mediocrity. By keeping the balance only means not ignoring any of the fields. And I said to keep all the areas in the right proportion, not all in equal proportion.

Some of the things can be used as a pinch of salt. We can follow the 80/20 rule. We can give 80% of the time to important tasks and 20% to the remaining. Besides this, we can follow the weekly routine to keep the balance between all the essential areas.

The subject matter of this chapter is very vast. I am writing a separate book on this subject. Presently, I have mentioned only a few of those aspects, just to make the achievers of greatness aware of life's true nature, essential for living a fulfilled life.

To sum up the key concepts, the number one thing everyone must know, we are here for a limited period of time, and nothing will come with us. The example of Alexander the Great, who expressed his last wish as: "*Bury my body, do not build any monument, keep my hands outside so that the world knows the person who won the world had nothing in his hands when dying,* "tells us the truth of life.

So don't take life very seriously. Treat this life as a big game, but remember the rules of this game are very stringent, universal, and eternal. At this very moment, though we can see and feel the world, in reality, there is nothing except energy. All the apparent things are all illusive. But we have to keep on living as long as we can witness this persistent illusion. Here some of you may think if everything is an illusion, then what is the point in living. Nature has created all of us, and there is nothing in the universe that has been created without purpose. So, find out your purpose. If you can't, then go and solve the people's problems. The problem you can solve better than others is the purpose of your life.

You need to be intellectual all the time. Finally, to live a fulfilled life, understand the importance of maintaining balance.

In the last concluding chapter, I will be reminding you of all the essential principles we have discussed so far very briefly. To make sure, you take away the right message.

Chapter 14

Recipe for achieving Greatness

Knowing the facts of life, the factor of impermanence actually expands your understanding, widens the perception of life, levels up your life for this big game. It takes you above the small, petty things of routine life. It helps you to think beyond your immediate future, expands your horizon.

It is said that if people remember you for few years after you pass away, then you are a mediocre person. If they remember you for 100 and more years, then you have done something good with your life. And if people remember you for more than 1000 years, then you are indeed a great person.

Now we know that our life is full of uncertainties. Several unexpected, unwanted things, incidents happen to us. If we keep on reacting to each event that is happening with us, our life will be like a boat without a sail, which keeps changing its direction according to the wind and will never know where it will land.

If only you have your life's purpose and have a clear picture of your destination in your mind, and know the direction, you can decide how to respond to these unexpected events. No matter what happens, you will invariably reach your destination. It happens because when you aspire to something intensely, the whole universe conspires to bring it into reality, as Paulo Coelho talks about in The Alchemist. It happens because you are connected with the entire universe at the fundamental level. Your thoughts and your mind are associated with it. Your emotions set the vibrations, and the universe reciprocates with vibrations of the same frequency. Therefore, you receive those things which you are holding deep in your mind, knowingly or unknowingly. So, set your goals.

You need to work on your self-image because that reflects your frequency, and the external circumstances are just the reflection of inside you. It would be best if you upgrade your thermostat, the concept Dr. Maxwell Maltz uses for self-image. What is inside is outside. Unless and until you change from within, make yourself big enough you can't receive anything worthwhile. It would be best to change your self-identity, which is nothing but your experience of your own self, which determines your responses, limits, and boundaries. Enlarge it. You can change your self-image as you wish by building the new habits that will make you the man of your dream. You can nurture your self-image by starting to live as the person you want to become right from now.

Now you know that nature has given each one of us the most powerful and immensely potential brain and the mind. If you learn how to use it, you can achieve anything, and that is what Neuroscience, Neuroplasticity, and Epigenetics are trying to teach us.

The most prominent quality of our mind is the ability to believe. Know this science of belief. This is the ultimate force on this planet that can sustain life and taking the lives in this Covid pandemic. Know the power of faith, which can make you or break you. Strong belief gives you inner strength and stability. It reduces internal resistance. You have to believe it before you receive it. Many of us may have some negative and limiting beliefs. But these are passed onto us by others, and we have accepted them as true. We can change them and replace them with new beliefs at any moment in time.

Remember, our brain is malleable and can be rewired with the help of strong affirmations. Care for your self-talk; that plays the magic. Always think positively and use the right words.

The other important quality of our brain is visualization. Visualize your future, design it, add the right emotions, and make your brain comfortable with the new you and your desired new life. Your subconscious mind is mighty enough that it invariably manifests your dream into reality.

Check your emotions every day because the quality of your feelings decides the quality of your life. Look for your inner focus. Where is it focusing? It attracts like a magnet, whatever it focuses. Set these two things right every single day.

Ultimately it is your character that decides your destiny. It is the foundation on which everything resides. Your success, happiness, everything sustains with the strong foundation of your character, and nothing worthwhile withstands when you compromise with it and with your values.

A healthy body and a sound mind are the means of achieving Greatness, are the source of all happiness, all fulfilment. Your health should be at your highest priority. Your health is the indicator of your balanced life. In her concept of **'The Whole Health Cairn**,' Dr. Lissa Rankin puts health on the top of everything, above the relations, career, finances, spiritual life, and creativity. If anything, or any one of these moves aside, the whole cairn crumbles down. It is the health, being on top, that gets affected first. So, bring and maintain balance in your life.

Finally, when you know this science of achieving Greatness and all the principles explained in this book, now when you have the right mindset and your intensity is high on fire, you are all set to march towards achieving Greatness.

Remember, **Consistency is more important than intensity.** The principles will work for you only when you take action on it, every single day. Action is the only key. Because with consistent actions towards your goal, everything falls at the right place. With momentum comes motivation, and with motivation, the mind stays positive, thinks positive. You start believing, and your self-esteem goes up. Your brain secretes the positive growth hormones. That helps you keep going.

Last but not least, remember, time is the biggest asset in this journey of achieving Greatness. Never ever waste it. Instead, invest it in building robust health, building strong relations, earning riches, creating abundance.

Time is your life, and it's running, and nothing on the Earth can bring you back the time that has passed.

The universe, the almighty God, has given you the wonderful gift of this life. Now it is up to you; what to do with it?

www.ingramcontent.com/pod-product-compliance
Lightning Source LLC
Chambersburg PA
CBHW070637220526
45466CB00001B/209